How to *Really* Lose Weight Without Dieting

By Anne Lyken-Garner

LIST OF CONTENTS

How to use this book

This is a step-by-step guide which painstakingly outlines how to lose weight naturally and sustain this weight loss for life. This programme is presented in a chronological order, so it's important to follow it in this way. This is about you, the reader, taking an active role in making this truly a personal effort.

Chapter one is the general description of the programme - giving the readers samples of how the guide works, what to expect, and a description of the tasks ahead.

Chapters two, three and four deal with different aspects of the first four weeks and introduce the basics of programme. These chapters go hand in hand to set the foundation of the new lifestyle.

The last chapter in this section outlines devious ways to prevent hunger from attacking, and points the readers in the way of healthy snacks rather than banning them altogether.

Chapter five offers vital psychological support and gives guidance on how to behave when temptation presents itself after the stepping stones have been laid. It provides the interim maintenance crutches between the introduction and the honeymoon period of the programme.

Chapter six starts week five of the lifestyle course. This entire chapter is dedicated to the issue of desserts because it's crucial to address this before moving on with the mind-training aspect of the programme.

Chapter seven is another interim chapter dedicated to the issue of food shopping. It's imperative that this be addressed because it has been revealed that our shopping trolley is a direct reflection of who we are and how we eat.

Chapter eight settles into the new lifestyle with the added bonus of a healthy and rational mind-set about food. It validates the safe period and steps up the commitment to the work at hand.

Chapters nine, ten and eleven reaffirm the journey and show how people who live healthy weight lifestyles maintain it permanently. It reveals the secrets of creating a different outlook about life and weight and gives the courage to keep at it.

Each chapter concludes with a timetable of what has gone on and what is to be undertaken next. Everything is laid out clearly in a simple format that shows what the journal (known as the H.I.T 'healthy ideal weight' journal) entries should look like. There is an ultimate task at the end of the programme, which will reveal to the reader their individual take on the entire system.

I've also included very large top and bottom margins, along with a couple of blank pages for your notes.

Kilo 1 – The Programme

Welcome to this step-by-step guide, which meticulously outlines how to lose weight naturally and sustain this weight loss for life.

This little handbook is a lifestyle-training exercise pointing you towards a healthy weight for your individual body shape.

The programme is presented in a chronological order so the tasks have to be tackled *and completed* one at a time if they're to work appropriately and make any impact to you or your body. Don't worry, we'll move as slowly and as naturally as possible.

You will not be dieting, nor will you be required to join expensive gyms. These are my two promises.

This road you'll endeavour to tread is the path of a more relaxed, stress-free journey. This voyage doesn't simply teach you how to lose weight, it conditions your body and brain to naturally hover at the weight which is ideal for you – not our mum's weight, or that supermodel's – yours!

If the body is yours, then the weight to which you aspire has to be just right for *you*.

You won't diet

Now then, we've said that you're *not* going on a diet. Why? It's one of the worst ways to lose weight because it imprisons you in a state of constant misery and hunger.

Having to relentlessly think about eating is the perfect temptation to drive one to stuff their faces full of sweet-tasting food. Instead of making you want to eat *less* – like it's supposed to – a diet encourages *stronger* cravings for food because it snatches away that which you've grown so accustomed to – a full stomach.

No one in their right mind wants to keep doing something which takes away one of their most satisfying pleasure.

Dieting, therefore, is self-punishment. It's denying you a relationship with one of your closest friends. No one wants to put their body under strain indefinitely, no matter how bad they feel about themselves.

This consequently, is why diets never last. This is the number one reason why we won't waste valuable time doing it.

Secondly, we don't want you to fall into that trap of self-denial (diet) because it takes away the nutrients your body needs by *not* allowing it a balanced diet.

It also shackles you into a miserable existence, which leaves you – and the people around you – holding your collective breath, turning blue and craving for the minute you could dive into a food pool again and get soaking wet.

Losing weight with this programme will be a pleasant, safe and healthy experience – something you would feel completely contented to sustain for the rest of your life.

If you expect this way of losing weight to take longer than fad diets do, you would be wrong. Why? Because you'll only have to do it once, and there will be none of the stop and start from scratch (over and over again) diets you've done in the past.

Of course, in the beginning weeks it *will* take time for the effects to kick in, but the overall result as you live this new lifestyle will be more than worth the initial patience output.

You will become one of the people you admire – one of the healthy weight people. We won't call them skinny, because you won't aim for skinny. Your goal is to arrive at your healthy, ideal weight - henceforth referred to as your H.I.T

Why would this work when other ideals have failed

- This book has been written by a former catwalk model (who worked in a poor country with none of the celebrity frills), who's at present a photographic model. I've experienced first-hand how difficult it is to stay in shape, especially after giving birth three times in as many years. After having kids the focus on healthy eating is no longer on yourself. And before you've had time to even brush your hair, it's time to get the kids washed and into bed. I know what a mother's life is like, but I've still had to stay in shape. I've been successful in doing both.

- This book is about getting back into shape without having to take time off to exercise and certainly without any dieting whatsoever. There is *no* pressure to put your body under duress, therefore no danger of life getting in the way of a separate exercise programme.

- The advice in this book is geared towards both obese people and those trying to lose only a few pounds. I'm not a fan of exercise, therefore, staying in shape for me has always been about finding ways to cheat the pounds so I didn't pile too much on in the *first* place. Anyone across-the-board will be able to benefit from the advice given here.

- This book guides you from the first spoon of losing weight and supports you through to the point of strength in maintaining not a weight loss programme, but a lifestyle free from the burdens of diet and punishing exercise. You'll have it to fall back on even when you slip up.

- This book does not tell you that snacking is wrong, instead it *points* you towards the right snacks. I reveal the personal secrets I've protected through the years, of foods you can use to trick your body into feeling full without gorging on large meals.
- This is one of the very few books on weight that says it's not a failing when you eat happy foods. *I believe that being able to indulge in happy foods is the very thing that's kept me on the right track health-wise.*
- One entire chapter is dedicated to the crucial issue of how you shop and another teaching you how to read your body's messages of hunger, thirst, or boredom – all of which send hunger signs to your brain.
- Your happiness while maintaining your new lifestyle is always paramount.

Well, this is only the start! Life and weight loss is to become increasingly easy to live with. Here is the key – sustainability. We want to be given something we can and *will* stick with. Right?

All you have to bring to this feasting table is a determination to make this big H.I.T last for the rest of your life, and keep a journal of what you're doing and what's going to happen next.

Kilo two awaits with the next step. Excitement is barely containable at the opening of this new door and contented life - a life in which dieting and food-related miseries are not welcome.

Are you ready? One step (one kilo) at a time is the way forward. *Do not start kilo three unless kilo two is conquered. Grab your journal and get ready to start your journey to a new life!*

Kilo Two – Begin With One Spoonful

Note: This chapter, along with chapters three and four, cover the first four weeks of the programme.

So here's your primary step. From day one, at every meal you'll serve yourself your regular portion of food then take one serving spoon of food (about four tablespoons) off the plate.

This means that eating on the go and picking food off the kids' plates – anything that means you can't truly gauge the amount you're eating – doesn't fit in with the programme. You will *have* to eat from a plate.

One serving spoon of rice, pasta, or spaghetti translates to the following:
Bread: divide into four and remove one piece
Potatoes: divide into four and remove one piece.
Pies: divide into four and remove one piece.
Salads: go crazy and chomp down the whole lot.

The reason for doing this little ritual of taking food off your plate is both psychological and physiological.

You will see the evidence of how little difference there is between what you normally eat and what you're eating now, so you won't feel like you're being deprived of anything.

One serving spoon is not a large amount, but it is less than you would normally eat. We're doing this in order to begin the process of shrinking the stomach. I should point out that the cheapest, safest and most lasting way to shrink this organ is not to have it diced and removed, but to eat less.

But would your body notice
Of course it would, it's being given a slightly smaller amount than usual in order to slowly adapt to needing less.

Starting your H.I.T life with one spoon less means that your stomach will be given ample time to gradually get used to it and get on with what it does naturally, start shrinking.

Because no dieting is involved, it will not go into shock of suddenly being deprived of the amount it's used to. For clarity purposes, this new amount will be called the *first shrink.*

Now, psychologically, you won't be craving for anything because in reality, you won't be missing anything.

What's next
After two weeks of getting used to the new amount, (don't rush it) you'll serve yourself this first shrink then take off another serving spoon. This newest amount will be called the second shrink.

Again, one serving spoon of rice, pasta, or spaghetti translates to the following:
Bread: divide the first shrink into four and remove one piece
Potatoes: divide the first shrink into four and remove one piece.
Pies: divide the first shrink into four and remove one piece.
Salads: go even crazier and chomp down the whole lot.

By now your stomach will be used to the first shrink, so you'll encourage it a bit further, but *only* by a negligible amount.

Remember that it's important to move slowly with this element of the programme as this is not all that you'll be doing, (see chapters three and four for making the complete basic H.I.T) do not take off more than one serving spoon at a time because you promised you won't diet.

Why? You don't need anyone to tell you that dieting will cause you to fail and pile on more weight in the end.

If it helps, place your original portion on one plate and the first shrink on another. On the first day of starting the smaller portions, take a photograph of these two plates and paste them in your journal.

If it suits you, you could keep a digital journal of the pictures of the foods, and a tape measurement of the size of your waist.

Lay the tape measurement on the floor, place a ruler or something with a straight edge at the size of your waist, take a picture and keep for your own reference.

Remember that you may not see any difference in the first two weeks. This is normal. However, you're now committed to a new lifestyle. Lifestyles, even for the rich and famous do not happen suddenly. Fads and phases come and go overnight, but we already know that.

Slow and steady is the key

Even in the world of celebrity, the most prevalent and popular faces, those who have staying power like George Clooney, Shirley Bassey and Tom Jones, are the ones who've started small and have built up secure solid foundations before climbing higher, hence the staying power in a world where not many ideals are born to last.

Slow and steady is the definitely the key.

THE TIMETABLE FOR YOUR H.I.T JOURNAL:
Hitting It – Day One, Week One

- Start a journal. You will need it for your most special task revealed at the end of this book
- Take photographs of your normal portion next to your first shrink. The first shrink is your original portion minus one serving spoon.
- Take photographs of a tape measurement of your waist size.
- Continue with first shrink plus the tips in 'kilos' (chapters) three and four – for two weeks.

Hitting It – Day One, Week Three

- Take photographs of your first shrink alongside the second shrink, which will then become your latest amount.
- Take photographs of your new waist size measurement (because the first sign of weight loss or gain is seen in the size of the waist).
- Continue with the second shrink for three weeks.

You will stick with this second shrink for weeks three, four and five. Your stomach will have shrunk quite considerably, but there are other things (that have nothing to do with eating) you've got to get on with for this to work properly.

Read on, as Kilos (chapters) three and four, whose activities run concurrently with this one, overflow with pride at the progress which has already been made – the sheer courage it took to make the change.

Remember to:
1.   Eat only from a plate.
2.   Follow the programme and cultivate the lifestyle slowly.
3.   Be patient and remember that the first two weeks are the settling-in period.

Kilo Three – Don't Over Exercise

This chapter runs alongside chapters two and four to help you achieve the introductory H.I.T. It covers the first four weeks of the programme.

Why not over-exercise? Simply because it's unsustainable

By now you're on your way with your first shrink. It's been great because the beauty of this programme is that it allows you to take your time to get used to a new lifestyle.

There is no sharp hook sunk into your soft middle, edging you to go forward when all you want to do is to taste something sweet on your lips.

Cutting down on food is only the *first* step. This goes hand in hand with giving the body physical activity.

Losing weight the gradual, natural way allows the skin to regain its elasticity because it's not suddenly been deprived of all the fat it's learned to support for years.

Physical activity will add to the attractiveness of measured weight loss because it will allow the fat to be slowly consumed, simultaneously converting it into muscles.

The largest organ of the body, the skin, also needs time to adjust to years of abuse. Like the stomach, it needs time to shrink, just as it needed time to expand.

Nevertheless, as busy people – many of us parents of small children – we really do not have the luxury to take time off for a separate exercise regime. Besides, we don't really like hard work and even if we did, there's tonnes of it waiting at home and at the office for us get stuck into.

Pace yourself

The weight loss programme for someone I know involved 400 sit-ups every day for five months, and a diet of *just* grapefruit. She rapidly lost a massive amount of weight, but because this self-torture was too cruel to bear, she quit altogether.

Needless to say, she regained all the weight she'd lost and a significant amount more for good measure. She's now doing a lot better on the H.I.T lifestyle, slowly getting there, but with a certainty of life-long success.

I eat three meals - and two snacks – a day and do forty sit-ups twice a week. I've done this for many years. The reason I am making this comparison is not to call your attention to my laziness. It's to point out that too much exercise will lead to a burn out and a frustration which will only culminate in quitting.

In the long run, extensive exercise will take up all your spare time and become a tedious chore. This is one of my promises, no heavy, burdensome exercise. Mind you, we didn't say '*no*' physical activity, did we?

Don't worry if you've never done sit-ups. I'll confess that after my third child in as many years, I couldn't even manage one.

My first sit up after having the kids was half a one. The next day I did one, the following day I did one again. By the end of the month, I was doing five sit-ups three times a week.

Now I can do fifty or more in one sitting but can't be bothered with any more than forty. Besides, I do them while the kids are having their wash and I have to get them all in before someone shouts, 'Mum!' from the bathroom.

A reasonable amount of physical activity will bring about a sense of achievement. It will be something you can stick to and most of all, something you can find the time to do as part of your new ongoing lifestyle.

I am not advocating that exercising is no good. On the contrary, I am all for it and do it regularly, but what's the point of taking on something which is too difficult and time consuming for you to remain faithful to?

There are several ways to take exercise without actually taking time off to do it

This one needs involvement from other people so while giving you examples of what you can do to get physical exercise, I'll show you how to get help from other people to make sure you stick with them.

Walking is a perfect example of getting your exercise in on the sly. Why not walk the children to school? If the school is too far away, leave five minutes earlier and park five minutes' walking distance away.

Assuming you're picking the kids up as well, this basic activity alone will give you twenty minutes of daily walking - ten walking back and forth to the car, twice. Not bad! It all adds up.

I get my twenty minutes of brisk walking (I speed up on the way back) every day merely by taking the kids to school. Now let's see what more we can add in.

When going shopping, instead of looking for a parking space near the door, find one as far away as possible near to a trolley bay.

This is an extra ten minutes or so of walking per week. In conjunction with our reduced portions, we're now taking gentle exercise as well. Add lots of fruit and water intake, and we're on a healthy path. This is good going.

Remember the aim is to take it slowly without dieting, but it is crucial to take all the points into consideration (and the order in which they are presented) and practice them for your H.I.T to be achieved.

There are several other obvious ways of getting exercise without taking time off to do it:

- Take the stairs - not the lift. Even if you do take the lift and ride it most of the way, come off two floors early and climb the two flights of stairs. This is just a start and can be increased as you become fitter and more confident.
- Try walking to a friend's house/book club/where ever you go for recreation.
- Take the kids to the park at weekends, not in the car but down the cycle path.
- Gardening is great for firming up those bingo wings.
- When the kids say, 'Play with me, Mummy', play hide-and-seek (not a computer game) or take them outside to play catch and go a bit nutty. Add this activity as ten minutes of your walking time.
- Swimming too, is a perfect way to exercise. And since most of us can do it, it's great to take up as a fun family outing. Take the kids to the community swimming pool on Saturday mornings and swim a few laps. This doubles up as family fun time and it's easy to forget that it's actually exercise.
- Walk the dog, or take up hiking as a pass time.
- Invest in a good bicycle and go riding with the kids (or just your partner) if you're looking for ways to spend more family time together. Your motto should be, if it's a mile or less, we can walk it. There is no reason to drive if the weather is good and you can walk there.

Getting help:

Tell your friends and workmates that you're banned from the lift. Say that if they see you heading for it, to close the door or order you to the stairs. This will give you support when you're weakening.

- Make a promise to your friend that from now on, every time you come over to visit you'll be on foot. She or he will no doubt expect you to arrive walking. Letting down yourself is private and does not give you the urge to keep your word. Breaking a promise to your friend is not something you will do lightly.

- Tell the kids that they're no longer going to the park in the car – ever. Give them permission to hide the keys if you ever suggest doing so.

- Ask friends who're already members of cycling or hiking clubs if you can come along. Give them permission to bug you until you join them. Who knows, you might really like the experience and want to go often.

- Seek people out who you know go running or jogging. Ask them how they train and make plans to go with them to see if you like it. Remember that patience is key, and so is pace. Don't go overboard and stretch yourself because there is only one natural outcome to making unsustainable commitments - quitting.

Later on, when we talk about settling into your new lifestyle we'll discuss how you can step up your physical activity without actually going to the gym.

Keep in mind that you're not dieting, and you're certainly not paying all that dough to join a gym because you know that the gym is not a magical place of weight loss – expensive place maybe, but not magical.

Once you've introduced physical activities into your everyday living, you're heading the right way. Let's see what awaits in Kilo four, when we'll see if we can answer the question, "What happens when my body wants food after I've eaten my second shrink?"

THE TIMETABLE FOR YOUR H.I.T JOURNAL:
Hitting It - Day One, Week Two

1.   Eating first shrink.

2.   Taking opportunities to get as much physical activity as possible.

3.   Eating from a plate to make sure that portions are correct.

4.   Staying positive and patient as you settle into week two of the H.I.T lifestyle.

5.   Upping water and fruit intake.

Kilo Four – Be Devious

This chapter goes hand in hand with the preceding chapters and covers weeks one to four.

So, by now we're on either our first or second shrink and we're introducing a manageable amount of physical activity into our lives. We're solidly building the endeavours of our H.I.T programme from bottom up. No fast track, no crazy unsustainable fads for us.

Now, that's underway, but I want to teach you a personal, secret trick. It will get better later, but for now, while still striving with your introductory H.I.T playing little tricks on your body is okay if you're doing them responsibly.

At this time you would've conquered the hard bit of actually making the decision to go with a healthier lifestyle. In the interim period you will need some crutches until you can stride through the journey all on your own. This is where the little tricks come in.

It is possible to fool your stomach into thinking that it's full

I know this to be true because I do it all the time. I love my body and won't do anything to harm it, and I've only been able to sustain this trick because it's a healthy one.

Drink a glass of fruit juice or ideally a fruit smoothie, and eat say a banana right before meal time. Your stomach is now partially full which means it won't require that much food.

Sitting down to eat your meal with a stomach that's not pining for food means that you won't actually crave that much of the calorie-rich dinners and lunches. You would've filled up their reserved places with heavy, satisfying, but healthy foods.

Many times we keep on eating long after we're full, not because we're still hungry, but because there's food left on the plate. If you go out to restaurants which serve large portions, it is okay to ask for two-thirds or half of it instead.

They won't mind the request as long as you're willing to pay the price of the food anyway. We've all heard of the saying, "Your eyes are bigger than your stomach." This is true.

Many times we keep on eating long after our hunger is satisfied only because our eyes can see how much food is physically there. *Sitting down to eat with a half-full stomach makes this temptation easier to resist. Not having that much food there in the first place doesn't present the temptation at all.*

It's also a good idea to have a glass of water or juice and some fruit just before you leave home to go out to eat. Not being famished means that you won't be tempted to order the largest meal on the menu.

If you don't like water and think juice is too expensive, squeeze lemon in water and top up with a piece of fruit and something naturally sweet (like raisins, or honey drizzled on pieces of apples) apart from biscuits. Again, the stomach is partially satisfied and the temptation to overeat is diminished.

It's good to fill up?

It is good to fill up on the things which are healthy – yet calorie poor. Eat less of the things which help the fat to bottleneck and finally fall out of creases in our bodies we didn't know were anatomically possible.

If the H.I.T is to be achieved, and it is, fooling your stomach into thinking you've already eaten is a fine way to do it. Nowadays though, your stomach is significantly smaller than it used to be. Becoming satisfied does not take as long or as much as it used to. Keep focused that you're doing this sensibly. The last thing you want to do is to re-stretch your stomach by gorging on anything you can find just because it's allowed.

Adult restraint is still required. Keep in mind that 'filling up' does not mean eating to bursting. It means eating until you're no longer *hungry*. There is a vast difference between the two, but it will take about three weeks' practice before you learn to identify the second one.

Remember this exercise does involve actual eating, as you're not going to be tricked into going on a diet.

As you begin the third week of portion control, when you're getting ready to start your second shrink, and have taken the pictures of both your first and second shrinks, do this additional thing.

Place beside the second shrink, a banana, a glass of orange juice (not fizzy drinks) and a handful of raisins. Take a picture of these and compare it with your first shrink. I think you'll see that the portions are significantly different, but if you take into consideration the three extra items of food which you'll be eating *before* the meal, you'll find that it's not that different after all.

The difference is in the calories! Why are we doing this? This is a vital question. The answer is that the first four weeks will be a settling in period into the new H.I.T lifestyle we've chosen. Support through these tender days is crucial, hence we will do all we can to help your body and you settle in with the least stress possible.

Once you get into weeks three and four where the actual food portion is significantly smaller, you'll realise that you can barely finish the smaller amount. At this point of feeling full – and here is a new sensation which you have to learn to identify – stop!

Success will only come if you learn to stop eating when hunger is satisfied

Yes, stop eating when you no longer feel hungry. There is no need to carry on after the glass of fruit juice or water, banana and raisins, and a small plate of food.

Your stomach is satisfied – this is good for the H.I.T. Stop eating. You don't have to empty your plate! This is the start of the new path and the certain sign that the H.I.T is ready to come.

When we were children we were told to empty our plates. Who's doing the telling now? We're adults and it's time to put our foot down and learn to read our body's messages.

The reason why stomachs stretch in the first place is because people eat more than they need. Imagine if you'd never eaten more than your stomach wanted, it would be the same size today as it was when you were thirteen years old!

If you can't finish the second shrink, don't push yourself. Put the plate down and walk away because it's time to prepare for kilo five.

THE TIMETABLE FOR YOUR H.I.T JOURNAL:
Hitting It - Day One, Week Three

- Take photographs of your first shrink alongside the second shrink, which will now become your latest amount.
- Take a photograph of your new waist size measurement (because the first sign of weight loss or gain is the size of the waist).

- Continue with the second shrink for three weeks. This means you'll be eating the second shrink for weeks three, four and five.
- Aim to sit down to eat – from a plate. Life will forgive you spending five minutes on retraining yourself to eat properly.
- Continue with physical exercise but get ready to step up as weight loss begins to even out.

Remember

- It's detrimental to the programme to skip meals at this point. This will set you back and encourage 'picking' or 'grazing' at odd times, increasing the amount you should be taking.
- Drink fruit juice or smoothie and eat a piece of fruit before eating a meal.
- Prepare to show restraint before you go out to eat by having something sweet like raisins or a banana drizzled with honey before you leave home.
- Ask for less food on your plate. Put less food on your plate so that the ingrained message of 'empty your plate' does not mean that you continue to eat after feeling satisfied (not stuffed).
- **The feeling of being stuffed warns you that your stomach is being stretched.**
- Keep drinking water and remember to monitor your thirst well. Thirst can send 'hunger' messages to the brain.

Kilo Five – Interim Support, Weeks Four and Five

This provides the interim support crutches from the introduction into the honeymoon period. This chapter concerns what happens from the start of week four to the end of week five when the H.I.T lifestyle should be settled into.

At this point we've already jumped the hurdle of the introductory phase of this H.I.T lifestyle. We've started and sustained both the first and second shrinks.

We've also made an effort to introduce physical activity into our everyday living at no cost at all. The hardest part is over. Now is not the time to fail.

What is H.I.T failure

You're now at the enjoyment stage. You're proud that you've kept on with this new lifestyle for so long, and have settled in somewhat.

You're at a mind-set of forward-looking and self-congratulation. Now that you've grasped and digested kilos one to four, *here are a few more things you should understand, especially if complacency starts to step in:*

Having an occasional biscuit or chocolate is not failing. Having to go to the extreme of banning happy foods forever, however, *that* is failing. But then again, so is devouring the whole pack!

H.I.T people eat chocolates, biscuits, crisps and various other fattening foods. The difference between Hitties (you) and those who fail, is that Hitties remove one or two from the pack, reseal it and eat them in another room.

The failers gobble down the whole packet, get the bits stuck to the corners of their mouths, then brush the crumbs off their laps in shame. As Hitties, we've practiced and now know how to read the signs when our stomach says it's had enough.

It is unrealistic to think that just because you've eaten two biscuits, 'I may as well eat the whole pack, because I've gone and failed again.' This is stupid talk. How does it make sense that because you've eaten two, you should eat the rest of the pack?

Does it not make more sense to say that now you've eaten two, it's time to put away the pack and save some for another day?

Later we will talk about what our bodies need and what they don't. We all know that we do not need biscuits, chocolate, or sweets for sustenance. We only have them because we can't resist the pleasure eating gives us.

Self-control is key here. If you find your old self returning when you sample your happy foods, here is what to do:

- Open the pack of (we'll use chocolate for simplicity sake) chocolate in the kitchen, remove a small portion of the bar.
- Reseal the pack and leave it on top of the cupboard in the kitchen.
- Eat your chocolate in a different room from where it's kept. Do not take the entire bar with you. As you know, this is a silly thing to do. Separating yourself physically from the temptation food is psychologically removing yourself from its hold on you. This will slowly break the cycle.
- Leave sweets (for example) in a box in the back seat of your car. You can't have them unless you're in the car and whatever you consume will have to be taken out of the box before you start driving (unless

of course you're willing to risk your life to get to your sweets).

- You should be able to work with these tips for now. If not, consult the chapter (7) on shopping. But I'm sure you can do this!

Lasting, healthy weight equals restraint and self-control

Remember you are not on a diet! You're grown-up and are perfectly capable of making your own decisions.

Therefore, you refuse to totally deny yourself happy foods because you know from experience that this will only make you want them more.

You're sensible enough to know that it is perfectly acceptable to have a little happy food – just like Hitties do. Since you're not on a diet, any food in small portions is okay, so the object of failing because of a stray biscuit or two is not an issue.

What happens if I pig out

What should you do if you decide to go on the rampage (and yes, this is a decision that you actively take, because large amounts of chocolates and biscuits don't just happen into one's mouth)? Unlike Robbie Williams or Brittney Spears we can't just pack our talented behinds off to rehab, we'll just have to dust the crumbs off our laps, wipe the corners of our mouths, and resolve to do better in the future.

So feel free to enjoy happy foods, just stop after a bite or two. This is the nemesis, fight and overcome! After week four (or thereabouts) you'll notice in your journals that your advancement has been steady.

You progressively lessened your intake of food, you'll soon learn how to snack on healthy options, your physical activities have been up-paced, and you're slowly beginning to need less food.

Solidify the new foundation

At this stage, you have to solidify this new foundation which you've built. You have to look at your notes and take stock of how your thought patterns about food and diet (the only banned substance) have changed, and look out into the future at ways in which you can make the permanent switch in your lifestyle.

Achieving H.I.T is not only about the tangible things like less food, more physical activities and lower caloric intake.

It is just as important to change the entire way you think about your body. We've talked about learning to identify when your stomach is telling you it's no longer hungry. This is crucial, and it may be impossible to achieve H.I.T without being able to identify this.

You also have to regulate the type of things you do, buy and consume, and the way you feel about them.

In the following chapters we'll discuss how this new H.I.T lifestyle requires definite self-control and a basic knowledge of nutrition.

You know that you're heading down the right path because for the first time, the weight you've lost is going to stay lost!

Regulating portions – check. Physical activity – check. Healthy snacks – we'll talk about. Not dieting – check! Not hungry or starving *or* craving for food – double check!

You have not failed, you've conquered! H.I.T is coming, so what more is there to iron out? Kilos six and seven are waiting just around the corner.

Just make sure that you're hitting all the foundation stones we've previously discussed before climbing onto the higher scaffolding of subsequent directives.

Four-Week H.I.T

At the end of the first four weeks you'll start to see a significant difference in your stomach requirements, and later we will talk about eating from a smaller plate but *not now*. Remember, this time it's not a diet (we don't like diets). This time, it's the new way of life that will nail it for good.

THE TIMETABLE FOR YOUR H.I.T JOURNAL:
Hitting It – Right Down the Middle
- Eating second shrink.
- Taking opportunities to get as much physical activity as possible.
- Getting up and brushing down if mistakes are made.
- Keeping focused while you prepare to hit the second part of the programme.
- Upping water and fruit intake.

Kilo Six – Do Snack

This chapter starts the second half of the programme. We're still at week five at this point, but have to stop to take care of an important issue before we move on.

Your journals should now be really underway. Remember that you need clear notes for your special task revealed at the end of this book.

You've got the pictures of both the first and second shrinks. You've taken the shots of your waist measurements and have watched with pride as it got smaller.

This is week five and along with the smaller portions and physical activity, you're ready for another little push.

At this point in time, your second shrink portion is still the one you're eating. You will continue with this up to the end of the week. However, in addition to maintenance, there is something small you need to do this week before we talk about healthy snacking.

This week's pressing task

It is time for you to knock one dessert off your week. So if you have one every night after dinner, you can now only have six per week.

If you had some four times a week, now is your chance to cut that down to three and so on. *You cannot move on to achieve your H.I.T unless you address the desserts intake. This is crucial! This is why an entire chapter is dedicated to it.*

One point to note, if you were having a dessert after every meal then I daresay, it's time to get rid of one entire day's worth of desserts. This is way too much and would *definitely* not help anyone to lose weight, regardless of how much physical activity you're now doing.

Remember if you never put it in, there will be no need to work it off. Soon popular desserts would be just an occasional thing for you. When this is ingrained in your thoughts, you've caught your H.I.T.

If a sweet taste after dinner is a must, try fruit with a drizzle of honey, tinned peaches and pears – or foods which we will discuss further in the following chapters.

Like the ex-smoker who yearns for something to do with his fingers long after he's given up smoking, if having something *extra* to eat after a filling, satisfying meal is important to you, try green tea with a drop of honey.

Not only will this satisfy your thirst and craving, it will work in your best interest because of its antioxidant properties. Tea is also something you can sip for a long time, providing constant work for the mouth to do.

The journal entry should reflect which dessert/s is going to be skipped and this should be maintained from this point onwards. The bottom line is that you have to train yourself to think of desserts as they actually are: extra, unnecessary, non-essential fattening foods you consume *after* a satisfying meal.

Do snack

Now that you're eating slightly less your body may feel a bit hungry. During the first and second weeks when you're serving up your first shrink it will be important to snack as often as you want, in order to keep the initial cravings at bay, and your reserve to conquer this strong. After this week the cravings, though still present, will definitely be less intense.

Is snacking healthy

The act of snacking is quite healthy. The unhealthy factor however, is *what* we snack on. A lot of people find that sitting in front of the TV cries out for a snack or two. Why not go ahead. Cut up two apples into fifteen or twenty little pieces (the *number* of pieces is important) and munch away. Apples don't do calorie counts.

Multiple pieces will take a long time to eat and with all the chewing involved, it is unlikely that you would want anything else after you've finished that marathon.

It is almost a chore to masticate for fifteen minutes non-stop. The crucial factor in this activity is that you're taking part in a most enjoyable pastime – eating, but that which you're devouring is calorie poor.

To achieve your H.I.T, you don't care if you're still eating like mad, in fact, we all love eating so bring it on! What you *do* care about is that you're satisfied and happy, but still able to approach the H.I.T by making wiser choices where food is concerned. You're also beginning to see the advantages of cultivating a mature sense of restraint.

If you're still hungry (and by hungry I mean bored) after the apple chunks, always keep a large stock of grapes at hand, these are great to snack on as well.

Try sunflower seeds and some of the other extensive ranges of healthy nuts on the market. Ethnic and Indian shops do a wide variety of savoury Pistachio nuts, chick peas, and cooked, seasoned lentils of every description.

I am aware that they are cooked in oil, but consider in one hand a basic and important food group like lentils and pulses, deliciously cooked in a bit of oil, and a large slice of cake in the other. No contest.

And while we're talking about cake, did you know that a glass of wine has the same amount of calories as a medium slice of cake? Well, now you know.

But I like sweet foods

For a sweeter delight, go for a couple of handfuls of dry (without the milk) breakfast cereal like honey-nut cornflakes. Just pop them in a bowl to snack on while you go about your business.

I find that a glass of water before a snack like this helps to fill me up too, and I often realise after I'd had the water, that I was actually thirsty and not hungry like my body had lead me to believe. So whenever you feel like a snack, try a glass of water before you start slicing and dicing. When your thirst is quenched, forget snacking and deal with the boredom in other ways.

Don't forget that fruit juices make a perfect snack as well, and are counted as part of the five a day portions of fruit and vegetables. At any rate, fruit is always good to have, whether we're hungry or not.

I don't envision that you will need the snacking crutch forever. Remember that this is just providing a way for you to learn what healthy snacking is. It's by no means a license to eat non-stop. As we said before, learning and understanding a new lifestyle means changing the relationship we have with food.

With the hunger sorted, done and dusted, let's see how your shopping can help you achieve your H.I.T in kilo seven.

THE TIMETABLE FOR YOUR H.I.T JOURNAL:
Hitting It – Week Five
- Eating second shrink.
- Taking opportunities to step up on physical activity.

- Getting ready to do the third shrink at the start of week six.
- Snacking healthily and responsibly.
- Drinking water first when the feeling of snacking hits.
- Cutting apples into tiny pieces for a lengthy snackathon.
- Upping water and fruit juice intake.

Remember

- **Important:** Boredom often presents as hunger. If you're having three meals a day there is no reason why you should be starving in-between them. The snacks I've outlined above are only a bridging method between your past and future lifestyles. You will find that once you've made the H.I.T you will not need these crutches anymore. If you do now and then, they're handy to fall back on.
- Desserts aren't needed for sustenance. They're extra foods we consume after we've *already* eaten. Extra pounds aren't force-fed into the body through meals but by fattening 'afters.'
- Cut food into tiny pieces when eating to quench your boredom.
- Have a glass of water before you snack. You may find that you don't need the snack after all.

Kilo Seven – Shop Right

This chapter takes you through week five and shows you the right way to shop for the life you're now ready to lead.

With the physical activities, second shrink (this is the last week of eating the second shrink), good food, lots of water, and a healthier attitude to eating and weight underway, we need to take stock at this point about what you're actually putting in your shopping trolleys.

This is your choice

We could've discussed this at an earlier point, maybe even to start with, but a lifestyle progresses in little steps and it wouldn't have done you any good if we'd plunged in with the drastic changes straight away.

The last thing I want to do here is to overwhelm you will all sorts of changes. First of all, it's important for you to make sense of *why* you're making these small adjustments, and for you to be willing to take the forward step in embracing them even before I suggest them to you.

Having the power in your hands to work these things out for yourself is the secret to changing your way of thinking. A H.I.T lifestyle then, gradually becomes more your choice and less my ideas.

Now that you're safely into the H.I.T kind of thinking, the time has arrived to make a change in shopping habits. This may be a bit hard for some people, but take it on gradually – as this is the only way it will work.

If you don't have it in the house/fridge, you can't eat it. This is why your shopping habits are extremely important to the programme.

Gaining or losing weight starts at the point of shopping

When you look into your packed shopping trolley, consider its contents a reflection of who you are and your lifestyle.

Here is an easy experiment: next time you go shopping look at the items in random strangers' shopping trolleys, and see if you can identify single people, cat lovers, new dads, people with a drinking problem, and people about to have a child's birthday party. It's easy, right?

In the same way, without seeing the shopper, you can tell a Hittie from someone who's not by the contents of his or her trolley. What picture does *your* trolley paint of who you are? Pay attention to it when you get to the checkout.

It's not too late then to chuck out the pieces of your reflection which you do not like. When you understand the direct relationship between your shopping trolley and your weight, you will find yourself paying more attention to what you put into it.

Leave it out if it's fizzy or fatty. Don't go overboard with low-fat and non-fat items. Our bodies need a little fat to achieve the H.I.T.

We all know that polyunsaturated fats like the ones found in olive oil are remarkably good for us and may even lengthen our life-span. Some people will go as far as to say that the fat in the food is *better* for you, than the poison put into it to remove the fat. If you're eating a balanced diet, you should be consuming all food groups *including* fat.

The bottom line is that if you like cheese, a little of it is good for you. Eating the whole block is obviously silly. No one needs fizzy drinks and diet varieties *do not* help us to lose weight.

They may not make us any fatter, but they certainly don't help us get lighter. Why would they? They are not healthy foods. You may think that this is too basic for us to even consider, but I've overheard two women in the supermarket deliberating on which fizzy drinks they should get.

Woman 1, "Get some coke for me, will you?"

Woman 2, "I thought you were on a diet."

Woman 1, "But it's only a drink. It's not like it's a bar of chocolate."

Woman 2, "Still. I think you should get the diet coke. It'll help you lose weight."

Woman 1, "Really? In that case, get me two cans then."

Diet varieties of foods *do not* help us lose weight. If anyone thinks this is so, you believe a lie. Granted, they may not actively cause us to put on any more weight, but they do not possess a magic mix of ingredients, which when consumed, lift the weight off our bodies. H.I.T means a desire, then action and dedication. Hence, you start with how you shop.

If you don't have it, you can't eat it

A lot of women tell me that they're unable to resist the chocolate mousse in the fridge no matter how hard they try. I naturally ask them if they do the shopping themselves, to which they normally reply, 'Yes.'

The obvious follow-up question is then, *'Why did you buy the mousse if you didn't want to eat it, and you knew that having it in the fridge would be a temptation to you?'*

Avoid putting yourself into situations like these. If you wake up in the middle of the night and go to the fridge to get something to eat (this is a really bad habit, but one that we will not discuss here), if healthy foods are all that's there, these are what you will *have* to eat. Otherwise, you may drink some water to quench your thirst and return to bed. If there are foods you know you shouldn't eat, don't buy them.

If there is an option of online shopping at your local supermarket why not do this for a few weeks while you settle in. It will help to go online just after your meal, so that psychologically your body isn't pining for food.

This means you won't be tempted to grab anything that looks good. After your body and mind are well into H.I.T focus, it would be safe to visit the supermarket again.

Just make sure that shopping is always done on a full stomach. This way, rather than beckon you, the fattening roasting chicken and chocolate topped cakes will not even take your fancy.

If you don't put it in, you won't have to work it out

Write the above sentence on the top of your shopping lists or purchase a stamp with these words on it and stamp it on all your lists. This is the belief I've always held in my H.I.T lifestyle.

I'm lazy when it comes to exercise. I am physically active but do not have the time, the funds, or the inclination to spend an hour every day at the gym working off two slices of cheesecake. In my book, this would be, 'What cheesecake? I never had any to begin with.'

For me this translates into not having to perform fitness bulimia on my body. *Why put it in if you don't want it there in the first place.*

Week Five's task

This week as you prepare to do your third and final shrink, there is one way to prepare your stomach for the news. This comes in the form of dropping another dessert in the week. If you really do not want your weight to plateau causing you disappointment and grief, you have to give your stomach another reason to shrink now.

This will be achieved by leaving out another dessert that you would've otherwise had. This omission is not just for this week, it's a part of the new lifestyle you're undertaking.

If you started with six desserts per week, you should now be on at most – three. This is the way forward. For the time being, substitute a piece of fruit or one of the sweet, healthy foods we discussed in kilo six.

Kilo eight beckons, while you take some time to sit down and decide what foods you need for good health and well-being, and which ones you merely want. The needs should be taken regularly, the wants – only seldom and in small portions. Make notes in your journal.

THE TIMETABLE FOR YOUR H.I.T JOURNAL:
Hitting It – Week Five
- Getting ready to start shrink three.
- Cultivating better shopping habits.
- Paying attention to the items in your trolley to make sure you like the reflection they give of your life.
- Staying with regular meals, eaten in plates.
- Snacking where necessary.
- Staying with physical activity, stepping up with walking, taking the stairs.

- You should've made up your mind about either cycling or jogging if you have the time.

Remember

Snacks are there if we need them, but with smaller stomachs, the bridging they provided should be needed a lot less now.

Kilo 8 – Time To Move On

This chapter covers weeks six and seven. It's the point at which we're expected to move on and be comfortable in the programme. You've H.I.T a new lifestyle.

It's time now – six weeks on, to move on to slightly more dedicated activity. It may help at this point to purchase a smaller sized plate from which to eat.

This way, the size of the serving is not so psychologically obvious. If you'd rather stay with the original plate to see where you've come from, this is okay too.

The third shrink

The time has arrived to take *half* a serving spoon off your plate – the third shrink. This time you don't need to remove the same amounts as you did before.

Half a serving spoon of rice, pasta, or spaghetti translates to the following:

Bread: divide second shrink into five pieces and remove one piece.

Potatoes: divide second shrink into five pieces and remove one piece.

Pies: divide second shrink into five pieces and remove one piece.

Salads: add more, go crazy and chomp down the whole lot.

This will be the final one – as we want to make sure we're getting enough food as adults to upkeep a healthy, active body. The only way you could venture into removing any more food after this is if your servings were giant-size to begin with.

I'll leave this up to you. Just keep in mind that you're not on a diet and don't want to starve yourself. Your aim is not to become skinny, but to achieve a healthy ideal weight (H.I.T) for *your* individual body. This means eating a healthy amount too. After all, we love food and hate exercise.

Just like you've done in the past, remove the required amount of food from your second shrink, and take a picture of the two plates for your journal.

If it helps, buy yourself a couple of new plates, which are smaller than the regular ones you're accustomed to eating out of. Psychologically, you will see yourself eating a full plate of food and it will also serve as a guide to how much your stomach requires, should you go away on holiday or eat at a friend's house (you can take your plate with you).

The idea is not to go back and stretch your stomach with large quantities of food. If you know any mother, you'll know that the second pregnancy shows a lot quicker than the first.

This is because the belly has already been expanded once, no matter how trim it became after the first baby was born, it's likely to stretch without much effort the second and subsequent times around. The stomach is the same because of muscle-memory.

Nowadays, you do not require that much help in terms of the fruit and nuts you eat just before the meals. But you should still have at least one fruit and a glass of pure fruit juice or water just before you eat. This is just to make sure that you're not starting on empty.

The 'keeps' and the 'dumps'

Stay with the healthy snacks and drink plenty of water. Again, you won't need the support of as many snacks as you did at the beginning. This lifestyle is not just about eating healthily, but also about eating less.

This was the aim from the beginning, right? By now the fizzy drinks should be mostly or totally gone from your body and desserts should've been significantly cut down. Over the next three weeks you will reduce your dessert intake to just one or two a week and no more. Fruit and fruit smoothies will take that 'sweet' place.

Try putting a spoonful of honey over fruit and feel them light up in your mouth. This is the perfect dessert - healthy and sweet.

Never mind the non-fat, genetically modified, preservative rubbish on the market. Go to the local fruit monger, get some fresh fruit, serve up with natural honey, and live large (though smaller in size than you used to be).

When the need for a dessert after each meal asserts itself, think of the mighty and gorgeous Angelina Jolie or the iron-buffed Brad Pitt. Would you say that they have a dessert after dinner each night?

You want to lose that 'levelling' feeling

Even though you've now lost a significant amount of weight, at this stage when there is a danger of it levelling out, it is important to step up a bit with the physical activities.

Remember that your body will soon get used to the physical activity you've been doing these past six weeks and with second shrink you've been eating. This is why it's necessary to now increase the pace.

You're not starting from scratch so it will be a natural progression from what you've already been doing. This makes it much easier to advance.

Instead of parking five minutes away do ten, now that your body has built up the expectation of a little walking. Instead of doing twenty minutes walking dropping off and picking up the kids, you'll now be doing forty.

This will give them a healthy twenty minutes of walking to and from the car. You of course will be going back and forth twice in one day – which gives you double the amount.

If you have to use a lift – even in the mall, you'll now take the stairs to three or four floors instead of the former two or three.

In place of two laps of swimming, you now do three. Maybe even consider joining a mother's group at the local church hall, doing aerobics or Pilates. Though joining up a group isn't necessary, it may be helpful if you're so inclined.

All the activity you need can come from walking, running and actively getting about your daily routine.

But if you think that working in a group could serve you positively, now may be the time to do so. Gym work-outs are not necessary in the least, as good cardiovascular, energetic exercise can be done just as well and better even, (certainly cheaper) outside of a gym.

If group work isn't your thing, there are hundreds of exercise tapes on the market, which are a lot less expensive than membership fees. Just buy yourself a couple and do them on your own.

Just make sure you see your doctor before you start, if they involve anything different from what you're accustomed to. It is a bad idea to jump into anything strenuous without first seeking medical advice.

Other organised activity

Pilates and Yoga tapes can help with relaxation and meditation. General aerobics, dancing, walking and running are more geared towards cardiovascular health and losing weight.

All different kinds of exercises including ones that relax you, those that make your heart race, and those that require you to exert energy, are necessary for overall health, building strength, and maintaining a healthy, constant weight.

Never forget that like an alcoholic, you'll always be affected by the over indulgences of your past. Like them, you'll always be prone to succumbing to temptations of filling up when your stomach's dial is saying 'satiated.'

Know this and be sensible about staying on the right track. It's up to you to decide to throw the former food-slavery lifestyle behind you, unshackle your mind, and embrace your new body and the new person you've become.

Meanwhile, kilo nine is there to uplift you while you invest in your new life and wait for the repayments you worked so hard to achieve.

THE TIMETABLE FOR YOUR H.I.T JOURNAL:
Hitting It - Day One, Week Six and Beyond

- Eating third shrink.
- Get rid of desserts and fizzy drinks.
- Buy some exercise tapes and work out to them on your own.
- Eat from a plate to make sure that portions are correct.
- Make attempts to do more organised activities.

- Pay attention to messages from your stomach.

Remember

Feeling stuffed or 'full to the brim' is a sign you're stretching your stomach again. Stop eating when hunger is satisfied. You have been able to identify this feeling for about three weeks now. Work with it!

Kilo 9 – It's Worth The Wait!

This chapter builds your stability through weeks seven and eight, at the point of reaffirming the direction of your journey.

Becoming a Hitty will take time. Weight will slink off gradually but there is a fantastic, positive side effect of this slow loss.

Your skin is being given enough time to gradually un-stretch itself. We've all seen those pictures in the magazines of young celebrities who were in a hurry to lose weight.

Crash dieting and liposuction don't give your skin enough time to keep up with what's happening to the rest of you and like the rapidly falling weight, your skin follows suit.

No one wants saggy flesh after losing weight. This is why doing it slowly is so important. Time gives your organs, especially our heart, stomach (the key to all this) and skin, good warning to catch up and get in line with the rest of you.

A good diet with lots of fruit and vegetables provide us with the right amount of vitamins and minerals to keep our skin healthy, elastic and attractive.

Crash diets leave it empty of the fat it's taken years to build up, not to mention – dry and wrinkly from the lack of nutrients we subject our bodies to when we go on diets.

Be prepared to wait, it is worth it

Perhaps no one will see your change for some time, but you can reward yourself by saving up the money you spent on desserts and sweets. Put this money aside and at the end of every ten kilos lost, buy something new.

It will be a treat when you naturally drop a size and have to buy a new set of underwear. This is one of the ultimate treats.

It may take others longer to guess what's happening, but that's alright. After all, your aim is not for the shocking presentation of a new body. It's a commitment to maintaining a new lifestyle for the rest of your life.

Your H.I.T will come, and when it does, unlike all the other times when you did the yo-yo, part-time games, this one will last. Why is this different? Simple!

This is not a diet that you'll do for three months, stop, then pile on all the weight again. This is a lifestyle so the 'showy' side of it will take longer, but it will *last* longer – forever from now on.

What a H.I.T life feels like

You will wait, and when the clothes don't fit anymore, you'll give them away. You'll get rid of the old reminders because the need for them will never arise again. Sure, it'll take longer for your friends to notice, and when they ask, "Are you on a diet?" you'll answer, "No, why do you ask?"

You'll tease them, but you'll tell them later on about this fantastic, new H.I.T lifestyle. You'll have to! It will be clear that you're different soon enough, not just in the way you look, but in the way you think about food.

The way your stomach feels satisfied when you walk down the street, *even* when you smell the neighbours' dinner cooking; the way you never gobble down treats in private anymore. *That* is the acid test.

Your thought patterns are different, which means you're no longer just following a weight-loss guide. *You* are the guide.

You're full until dinner time these days, and that's because you have a snack between meals. Not those fast-food preservative-saturated rubbish you used to crave, but nice food, fresh food that makes you feel good and proud (not guilty) after you've eaten them; food you have to chew and concentrate on eating; foods like cherries and grapes and nuts that burst with flavour and sweetness when you bite down on them.

Your mouth waters for this kind of food. You no longer have to *pretend* that you eat only healthy foods by showing off a hated salad in public, then devouring and ripping the life out of a king-sized burger when no one is watching.

There is no pretence anymore. What you eat in public is exactly the same as you eat on the sofa in the evenings while watching your favourite programme.

Where your H.I.T mind is

You don't aim to be skinny and unhealthy. Your H.I.T gives you energetic, happy health; the kind that ensures you receive all the nourishment you need and none of the fat, fizz and rubbish you don't.

The best thing about waiting for your H.I.T is that you're happy. You're never starving, yet never feasting on fast-food.

You're never craving because you haven't denied yourself food, yet you're no longer stuffing it down when no one is watching, feeling guilty for once again cheating on your diet. Hey, that's because you're *not* on a diet!

You feel a lot healthier now because your energy levels are getting higher. Your body is more used to physical activity because you're taking steps to make sure you do them.

Now you're ready to take control and be dedicated to pressing forward into Kilos ten and eleven. Kilos one to eight have been firmly set as your new lifestyle.

THE TIMETABLE FOR YOUR H.I.T JOURNAL:
Hitting The Old Life to the Curb

- Maintaining shrink three, healthy snacks, and physical activity.
- Making a list of physical activities undertaken and noting how they can be increased.
- Making notes on weight-loss and inches lost from waist measurement.

Kilo 10 – Learn to Read Your Body's Messages

This chapter reveals what should be happening during weeks eight and nine as the passage through your new life gets more enjoyable and feels more natural. It also recaps and verifies the steps that should be taken for the H.I.T to be made.

The journey so far

You've been eating smaller portions for eight weeks and have been successfully sustaining this.

You've been drinking more water and eating a bit of fruit just before your big meals so that your stomach starts on 'full' and is not looking forward to a total devouring devastation.

You have a better thought pattern about food - you don't think crazy thoughts like you used to. After all, you're not on a diet.

There is no need to crave after anything because there's nothing missing. Well, apart from the guilt of overeating – that is.

You do way more physical activities than you used to. You make a point to park far from entrances so that you can walk more often.

You get off the lift three or four floors before yours so that you could walk the rest of the way. You feel a lot better since you're shopping right.

Whenever the urge to snack hits you, you give in to it, but instead of reaching for the biscuit tin you have chopped fruit or nuts.

Watching television is no longer a guilt trip for you since you sit down with increasingly smaller bowls of healthy, satisfying chopped apples/grapes, nuts, dry breakfast cereal and so on.

You don't eat when bored anymore. That's your yesterday – your past. It is at this point, eight weeks down, when you've started to see real results that you'll be tempted to rush on and take big steps. Don't!

Remember that whatever weight you've lost in a matter of a mere eight weeks, will be multiplied by itself in the years to come. Yes, years.

Weight will be lost regularly with this new lifestyle because there is no quota – no time limit before the bulging starts again.

There will be no bulging - no gorging. Slow, steady steps are the key to the H.I.T. You've worked successfully so far and will achieve in the end. Do not lose sight of this. Before you take further steps at this point there are a few factors which you have to properly digest.

Am I hungry or just thirsty

As I mentioned before, it is important that you read our body's messages correctly. Sometimes you feel 'hungry' because you're a little dehydrated.

What the body is actually 'hungry' for is water, but somehow you read the signal incorrectly and dump food down your throat. Wait. Your stomach is smaller now but there will always be a fat stomach somewhere in there lying dormant, waiting to burst out.

Again, try drinking water first when you feel hungry, especially if it's not meal-time. *It's normal to feel like eating something sweet when you're thirsty.* This is exactly what happens after meals.

I grew up in South America and we were always taught as children that it was good to sit down to eat with a glass of water. This sounds like an old wives' tale but it's not. Having a bit of tepid water after a meal settles it down and takes care of that 'I need something sweet' desire, because you're no longer thirsty.

It is vital that you choose water over fizzy drinks and squashes to quench your thirst. Water is pure, natural and calorie-free. Never go without it. Remember not to substitute water for a meal (*you're not on a diet*). However, if you've just had a balanced meal, water – not a dessert – will wash it down nicely. Water, water, water.

Am I hungry or just bored

Again, if you're in between meals and hunger strikes, it may be that you're just bored. The brain desires to be stimulated at this point, but is the stimulant food? Hardly ever.

Try rekindling hobbies, do something for someone else, volunteer, read a book, have a glass of water. If you are bored, eating is definitely not the way to go for the H.I.T to take effect. As you're aware, food is merely *one* of the many desires we have as humans. Consequently, not all human needs can be met by eating.

You need to find out what is actually lacking in your life and work towards ironing out that.

Many times we turn to food to fill us up but the hunger we're desperately trying to satisfy does not emanate from our stomach. This is the reason why the craving isn't satiated no matter how much we eat.

Sadly, you will never be satisfied if your drive for eating is psychological. Only physical hunger can be satiated by putting food in your stomach.

The stomach is a relatively small organ so where is all the hunger coming from?

Am I still hungry or am I finishing the food just because it's on my plate

Now that we're adults, there's no one around to say, "Empty your plate." So why do you still feel you have to? Learn to read when the stomach is saying it's full. When it is, it's perfectly fine to stop eating. Even wild animals do.

It's still fine to eat out

Since you're not on a diet, it's still fine to still eat out. This is an enjoyable affair, why should you punish yourself by not doing so.

Just cut down on the amount of times you do. It is perfectly acceptable to ask for a reduced portion if you have prior knowledge that the servings are big. If you don't, either ask for a doggy bag or leave the rest on your plate.

Your smaller stomach now requires less food. It's not worth spoiling all that hard work with one night out. Keep in mind that fish and seafood dishes are smaller and healthier than the chicken and steak varieties.

The foods you need, versus the ones you want

I am not going to list the foods our bodies need to stay healthy – we all know them. If we have a bit of carbohydrates, some vegetables and meat/pulses on our plates, we're heading in the right direction.

Don't stop eating meat, but instead of making chicken stew (for example) with just chicken, cut down on the amount of chicken you use in one meal by adding tinned, ready-cooked peas and pulses, as well as tinned, chopped tomatoes.

It'll taste better and you'll have a balanced pot of warm stew with pulses (a needed food group we neglect).

It's a good idea to mix in tinned pulses and tomatoes to almost anything you cook.

You don't have to take extra time to cook pulses if you use the tinned variety. They increase the amount of brew significantly, and cooked in this way, you (and your children) don't even have to taste them. The important thing is that you include them in your diet.

Curries can have less meat and more vegetables. This is another great way of disguising vegetables if you don't like them that much.

When you've fed these balanced meals to your body it really does not require topping up with a dessert - even more food.

Simply put, after a balanced meal there is no need to bring out the sweet food. I am not saying banish these foods for eternity. What I am suggesting though, is now that you're well into your H.I.T lifestyle, it is imperative to accept that desserts aren't foods we need, they are fatteners we want.

This food group is the one which fattens us most of all. These are the culprits you *must* keep your eyes on, because they are the ones that will hurt you the most.

It would've been crazy for you to even consider this at week one, but now you've been H.I.T from head to toe, desserts have to be checked in order to continue.

THE TIMETABLE FOR YOUR H.I.T JOURNAL:
- Eating shrink three amount.
- Drink water when you feel hungry or feel the need for sweet.
- Lessen the snacks because with a smaller stomach you don't need that much anymore. Make use of the healthy options when you need to.

- Maintain a steady amount of physical activity and step up from where you started.
- Walk wherever and whenever you can.
- Take the stairs and park away from entrances.
- Use healthy-lifestyle exercise tapes at home.
- Shop right.
- Cut desserts to one or at most, two per week.
- Ask for smaller portions when you eat out.
- Substitute water and fruit juices for fizzy drinks.

Kilo 11 – What do I do With the Rest of my HIT Life?

This chapter covers week ten and onwards.

Well, this is certainly not the end

In fact, it's the beginning of a new pathway – a new life, a life not taken over by food and cravings of food, but one which is disciplined, active and clever.

It is easy to enter into a plateau, to become the person who gets tired of routine and discipline and reverts to the simplicities of satisfying craving after craving.

But you see, you've *been* there, and to go back would be like a dog returning to its own vomit. This is the last thing you want. As a matter of fact you don't want this at all.

So how do you continue in this new life you've donned? Just remind yourself why you want it.

You're proud of the fact that you now like yourself and are secure in what you've achieved. Not only have you changed the way you look – for good, but you've overhauled the way you think in private about food. This was the highest achievement of all.

Forward march

Now you've set your sights to the future and know that food will no longer take over your life. You understand that you'll always be susceptible to the temptations of food.

Rather than doing it naturally, you'll continually have to *make the effort* to think like a Hittie, but armed with this knowledge, you are strengthened to beat it.

Food had become a sort of drug, quite like alcohol is to alcoholics. Once an alcoholic stops drinking he or she continues, not so much to struggle, but to understand why they previously needed to fill a hole in their lives with a substance.

Once this acceptance is reached, it becomes easier to identify the signs of this need returning. If one can recognise the signs, one can prevent the dependency starting all over again.

And speaking of alcohol...

Binge drinking and glasses of wine after meals have no place in a Hittie's life. Your body has been transformed to need natural, healthy food and activities that are good for it. In terms of calories, one glass of wine is equivalent to a chunky slice of cake.

As you only have one, or at most two desserts per week, you can see that alcohol is to be kept at a minimum.

A large amount of alcohol as you know, is detrimental to your health because of the way it corrodes your organs – especially your liver. But not only this, alcohol drains your skin of its moisture, lessening its elasticity and youthfulness. If this is not enough, it makes you fat.

You have gone through a total re-conditioning of what you thought your body needed in the way of what you consume.

You now understand that you never actually needed half as much as you thought you did – either with food or alcohol. If you haven't decided why this was so, then you need to stop and do so now.

Old habits die hard

As a writer sitting at home for hours banging away on my computer keys, it is easy to go to the fridge and get food, but as we discussed before, if you don't buy it you can't eat it.

After a good breakfast followed by a banana for energy, I have an apple for my morning snack. I make sure that I'm drinking enough water throughout the morning.

There are several ways of reminding oneself to do so. One can fill up a bottle and finish it by lunch time, or drink after each natural expulsion of water.

If we drink only at meal times we may not be getting enough water, but please do not go overboard with this either. You want to keep your vitamins and mineral *inside* your body, not wash them away.

At lunch I take a break and cook noodles or rice with stir fry. I do a different flavour of stir-fry every day, using various vegetables mixed with tuna, sardines, or a little meat.

It's a small meal but it's totally balanced and tastes fabulous. Couscous (I have to use couscous made from maize) and omelettes are also wonderful, fast, tasty meals that can be mixed with anything.

This is all my body needs in the middle of the day, but I always have a mug of fruit smoothie with my lunch.

This makes it extra special and totally enjoyable. I look forward to it, and once I'm done, I'm totally satisfied; firstly because it's a good, tasty, balanced meal. Next, because my mind is made up that I am, and lastly because my stomach now only requires a small amount of food.

Notice I don't have a dessert. The fruit smoothie is more than enough for a sweet taste.

If I'm hungry mid-afternoon I have a rice biscuit with almond butter.

This takes me all the way to dinnertime when I have a serving of fruit, or a handful of dried fruit, and a glass of fruit juice or water. This is part of my dinner so the food on my plate is not a large amount. I have some warm water or peppermint tea to quench my thirst after dinner.

At no time am I starving or craving. If I feel hungry, which is a perfectly genuine request for the body to make, I have a glass of warm water, and if I *still* am hungry, then I have nuts or fruit.

Whatever you do, don't skip your meals because all the training you've done over the last few weeks will be in jeopardy. Make healthy eating your habit – and you know what they say about habits.

Our conclusion

In the ten previous chapters we covered a step-by-step guide of how to get to one's healthy, ideal weight (H.I.T).

We concluded that being thin is not necessarily healthy, and that the most important thing about getting fit is working out what weight is perfect for you and you alone.

It's now time to go over these points to make sure that you've done what you're supposed to do to stay new, and you understand *how* to make this lighter, healthier person stay that way (and progress) for the rest of your life.

This chapter's task is most important. This task is what makes the H.I.T lifestyle individually and ideally yours, and not based on anything I've said in this book.

You now have to go over the notes you made in your journal and point out each step you took towards this place in which you now stand.

Decide what worked for you and why it did. Decide what was not so hot and why not. I'm handing this over to you.

Now make up *your* own ten-week plan for the next couple of months or so. Make yourself follow it word for word, step by step.

Now you know how to draw up blueprints, you need to make one based on what worked for you in the past, that's going to work for you in the future. Keep your notes with you and make them guide you through your new life. **This is now all about you. Go ahead and write your own script!**

NOTES

63

NOTES

www.ingramcontent.com/pod-product-compliance
Lightning Source LLC
Chambersburg PA
CBHW070614290526
45790CB00002B/905